Dr. Lyle BULLER & Brian WILKES

Chinese Herbs
for
Martial Artists

中國藥材
武術表演

by Brian Wilkes
with Dr. Lyle Buller, NMD

ISBN-13: 978-1497542624
ISBN-10: 1497542626

DEDICATION

To the late Dr. Lyle Buller, NMD.

Thank you for sharing your training and experience with the world, and for allowing me to present it in a way that has helped thousands to heal.

Rest in Peace.

Chinese Herbs
for Martial Artists
中國藥材武術表演

DISCLAIMER

IMPORTANT: **For educational purposes only.** This information has not been evaluated by the Food and Drug Administration. This information is not intended to diagnose, treat, cure, or prevent any disease.

This information is **folklorical** and not intended to be medical advice. It is based on historic usages of plants in Asian cultures. It is not intended to be a medical guide. Nor is this book intended to be an alternative to any necessary medical treatment. If you need a doctor, see a doctor.[1]

Contents

Dit Da Jow: 跌打酒 Iron Strike Wine

The Magic Healing Potion You Can Make at Home

For one-half the cost, and in many cases twice the effectiveness, you can make a healing liquid that is better than anything available at the store.

Dit da jow, or "iron strike wine," is common to many forms of Chinese martial arts. Or to be more precise, the concept *of dit da jow* is common. Exactly what a *dit da* formula is supposed to do and how it works elicits as much opinion and heated debate as how to distill the perfect Scotch or cook the ultimate chili.

A Westerner can make some sense of the apparent confusion by realizing *dit da jow* is a generic term for a family of herbal preparations to be used in conjunction with iron-palm training. Iron-palm training itself has been the subject of much contradictory information in the West; for our purposes, it is the repeated striking of a bag of iron pellets, pebbles, or beans to strengthen the muscular and connective tissues of the hands and to teach the student how to direct chi into the target.

A pre-practice *dit da jow* must loosen muscles and connective tissues in the hands, so chi can flow through the hand during the striking. This type of formulation often is applied as a hot oil or as a pot of hot liquid in which the hands are soaked.

A post-practice *dit da jow* must heal any damage that has occurred during iron-palm training. Since proper iron-palm training should result in nothing worse than occasional bruising, this formulation is not geared to more serious damage such as bone contusions or sprains. Iron-palm training is not for "hardening" the skin or knuckles, so don't look for something that will build up calluses. In fact, in classical arts calluses are regarded as the symptom of an inferior martial arts.

A between-practice *dit da jow* is a general strengthener, and is often taken orally (*yao jow*, medicinal wine, or *yao pian*, pills).

Each school or sifu has its own "secret recipe" for *dit da jow*, since as the masters say, "no *jow*, no power." Featured here is the recipe of Dr. Lyle Buller, a chi kung practitioner and doctor of naturopathy who recently has moved into the Pine Barrens, a wilderness area of southern New Jersey. He finds the wetlands a rich source of botanical materials.

Dr. Buller's interest in Chinese herbal medicine dates to his student days at New York University, near Manhattan's Chinatown, where he worked for the president of the Chinese Herbalist Society of New York, who later became director of the Oriental Medical Institute of Hawaii. Dr. Buller also practices *tai chi chuan* and Vietnamese freestyle kickboxing. To understand the action of a *dit da jow*, Dr. Buller says you must first understand the basic anatomy and functions of the soft tissues.

"This formulation is based on what happens to your body when you get a bruise," he notes. "There is a layer of energy just beneath the surface of the skin and external fat, called the *wei chi*. It is this energy that protects you against 90 percent of external injuries, and can be thought of as roughly analogous to the lymphatic system. In Chinese medicine, it is this system that is strengthened with chi kung breathing exercises, and advanced exercises like 'iron shirt' or 'golden bell cover.' If your chi is strong, even a knife blade can be deflected (but not stopped) while you move out of the way or prepare a counterattack. A bruise is a gap in this protective layer of *wei chi*. This is more serious than it appears, since the gap can be a doorway for what Chinese medicine calls 'evil pernicious influences.' "

Although it sounds pretty spooky, "evil pernicious influences" can be understood as neurological disruption or a reduction in general immunity. The term comes from the Chinese belief that if the pores open too far, a "bad wind" or "wind attack" can get into the body.

"When you get a bruise, you also have blood stagnation," Dr. Buller notes. "Because of ruptures in the capillaries arid smaller veins, the blood pools in surrounding tissues where it stagnates and turns purplish-black. When the. bruise turns red a few days later, it's because the stagnation has broken up and fresh blood is beginning to move into the area again, and that new blood flow helps rebuild the injured cells."

Blood stagnation leads to swelling, which closes off other blood vessels, can damage nerves, and in extreme cases, can tear the skin. In Chinese medicinal theory, it also closes off chi vessels. Each of these effects can obviously lead to other problems.

A post-practice *dit da jow* must, therefore:

- Remove blood stagnation (this is where most formulations fail);
- Remove chi stagnation;
- Tonify the blood (return blood components to a proper balance);
- Tonify the chi (correct both direction and "volume" of chi flow) and: .
- Reduce pain to reduce involuntary reflexive muscle tension and spasms. Dr. Buller quotes the old Chinese maxim, "Chi moves, blood flows; blood moves, chi flows."

Another function of the *dit da jow* is bringing chi to the surface (*wei chi*) from deeper in the body (*ying chi*, the chi that circulates through the 12 meridians).

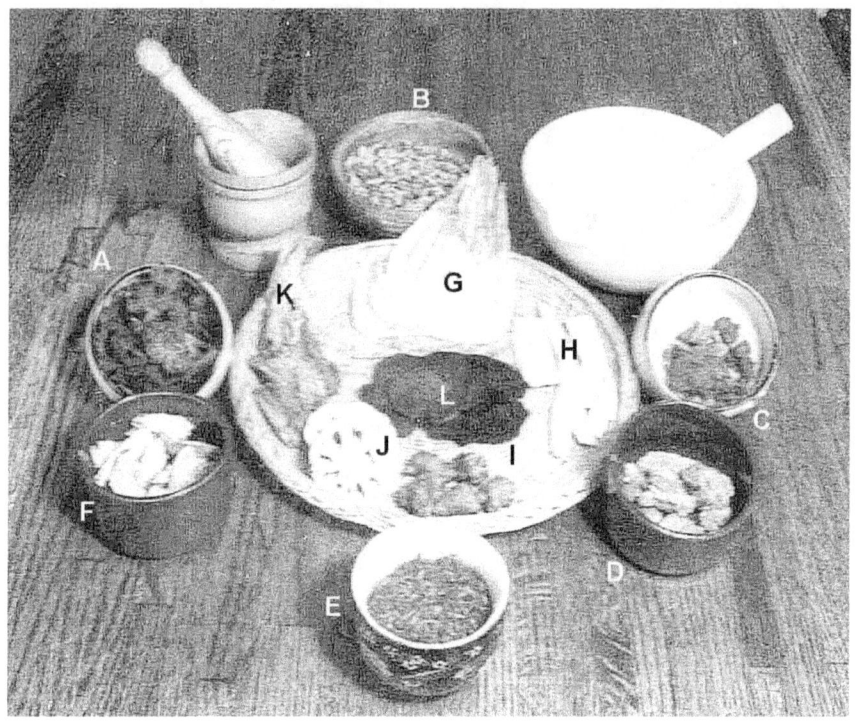

A Chuan Xiong -River parsley
B. Kuei Chih -Cinnamon twigs
C. Mo Yao -Myrrh
D. Ru Hsiang -Frankincense
E. Hung Hua -Safflower
F. Kan Tsao -Licorice
G. Tang Kuei Mei -Dong quai "tails"
H. Pai Shao -White peony root
I. Tien Chi -Pseudo-ginseng
J. Lien Tzu -Lotus root
K. Huang Sun -Skullcap root
L. Sheng Dl Huang -Rehmannia

Ingredients :

1. 桂枝 *Gui Zhi* (Cinnamomum cassia) cinnamon twigs

The wood and bark elevates blood temperature locally, and removes chi stagnation. This is not the dried, powdered cinnamon bark used in cooking, but the whole twig.

2. 生地黄 *Sheng di huang* (Rehmnannia glutinosa, raw)

A resinous compressed root, rehmannia is a blood tonifier. Some herbalists confuse this plant with American foxglove, which contains digitalis. This is a different plant. Do not substitute foxglove, since the digitalis can stop your heart. Rehmannia is sold in both raw and steamed versions, which have different properties steamed varieties which have different properties. We are using the raw (sheng). It resembles a flat patch of tar.

Cinnamon warms the blood and expels "evil pernicious influences", while rehmannia begins to cool the blood. With too much heat or cold the blood begins to stagnate, so these two work together to form a balance.

3. 藕根 *Lien tzu* (Nelumbo nucifera) lotus root

The dried root of an aquatic flower, lotus rebuilds damaged veins and capillaries, stops internal bleeding, reduces pain and swelling. In cross-section, the dried root resembles an eight-spoked wagon wheel, which is one reason it became the symbol of Buddhism, with its Wheel of Dharma representing the Eightfold Path. For Westerners, the resemblance is more to wagon wheel pasta. This has been known to cause confusion when a bag of the root is mistakenly bought, taken home, and boiled - and somehow, just doesn't smell like macaroni!

4. 田七 *Tien chi* (Gymnura pinatifida or Panax notoginseng) tien chi or pseudo-ginseng

The nutlike node of a root that grows on the edge of cultivated fields, *tien chi* ("field seven") reduces pain. Sometimes called *"tien chi ginseng"* or "pseudo-ginseng," this root is one of the most celebrated herbs in Chinese medicine. It's been "discovered" in America and recently has become something of a fad. Because of its scarcity, it is the most expensive of the ingredients. Tien chi stops internal bleeding, breaks up blood clots, lowers blood cholesterol and removes cholesterol deposits from artery walls -all of which come under the head-ing of "removing blood stagnation." *Tien chi* also has its place in European history; according to some sources, it was this root that the Russian mystical priest Grigory Rasputin used to treat the hemophilia of young Prince Alexei Romanov.

5. 黄芩 *Huang sun* (Scutellaria baicalensis) skullcap root
Also called *pan chih lien*, scutellaria reduces pain and swelling, and detoxifies the blood. Chinese medicine uses the root and stem; a Western herbarium's scutellaria might instead be dried leaves. Be sure you get the right ingredient.

Lotus "combats rebellious chi" in the veins. "Rebellious chi" means energy that is moving in an erratic or unbalanced way; this can be caused by a chemical disruption (drugs, alcohol, poor diet) or from not allowing the blood and chi to flush out the system (insufficient rest, returning to practice too soon after an injury). Pain comes from stagnated or "rebellious" chi and blood. These three painkillers help this, as will the three blood invigorators to follow. Scutellaria further reduces swelling; tien chi breaks up stagnated chi and congealed blood.

6. 红花 *Hung hua* (Carthamus tinctorus) safflower
A dried flower similar to saffron, used in dyeing as well as medicine, safflower removes blood stagnation and reduces pain. It's commonly sold in Chinese pharmacies as "red flower oil" tincture.

7. 乳香 Ru Hsiang (Boswellia glabra) frankincense

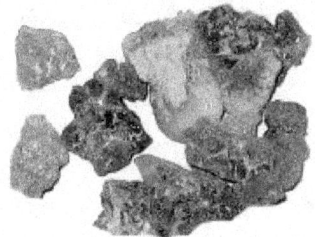

A resinous extrusion from a Middle Eastern vine, this was introduced to China by the Mongols. The Chinese name means "milk sweet," which gives some idea of the fragrance. Frankincense removes blood stagnation.

8. 没药 Mo yao (Commiphora malmal) myrrh

Another important herb from a vine resin, myrrh has a more bitter fragrance and is often used in conjunction with frankincense. The Chinese name includes the word *yao* ("medicine"), showing the importance of the herb. Myrrh removes blood stagnation.

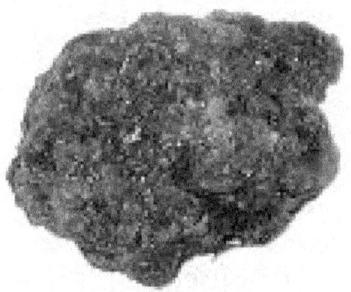

Although both come from vine resins, myrrh and frankincense behave differently. While frankincense looks like transparent pebbles or amber, myrrh looks like wood chips. In bulk states, they can look almost alike. If you're confused, try this test: Apply pressure with your finger or a hard object. Frankincense tends to be hard, and crumbles into grains. Myrrh is softer, and flakes apart.

9. 川芎 *Chuan Xiong* (Ligusticum lucidum/wallachii) river parsley, hemlock parsley

A tuberous root common to the Chinese highlands, this detoxifies the blood and also removes blood stagnation.

Safflower increases circulation by affecting mainly red (oxygenated) blood. Since the lotus has already repaired the small veins in the skin, the safflower increases red blood flow. If this order hadn't been followed, there would be more stagnation.

"A bruise is like a swamp: prepare the drainage and remove the water between the reeds to restore the environment."

Red blood near the surface of the skin travels between cells instead of in vessels, guided by chi; hence the metaphor. Myrrh, frankincense and *chuan xiong* circulate blood between cells to begin healing and removing stagnant blood.

10. 甘草 *Kan tsao* (Glycyrrhizae uralensis) licorice
One of the most useful plants in any herbal, licorice is a chi tonic, removes chi stagnation, opens all 12 meridians, purifies the blood, reduces pain, lowers body temperature, and detoxifies the effects of other plants in a formula. The Chinese name means "sweet grass," and the sweeter the licorice, the more effective it is. Unlike the American *glabra*, which tends to be a tight brownish wood, the Chinese *uralensis* has a porous yellow wood. Either can be used in this formula.

11. 当归 *Tang kuei* (Angelicae sinensis) dong quai
The second most abused root in Chinese medicine (after the ubiquitous ginseng), *tang kuei* tonifies and nourishes the blood and promotes healing of broken blood vessels. Since tang kuei is so popular, thanks to its undeserved reputation as a cure-all, it's also expensive (except for Korean *dong quai,* which is very weak and usually sold as a powder). Instead of the fist-sized whole roots, martial artists often prefer the fingerlike "tails" that branch off the main root. These also are much cheaper. Dried whole *tang kuei* sometimes is mistaken

for dried shell-fish, mushrooms, or white chocolates. Sliced crossways, they are sometimes mistaken for dried jellyfish!

12. 白芍 *Pai shao* (Paeonia albiflora) white peony root

Grown in semiarid climate, the pinkish-white peony root nourishes and tonifies the blood. It also raises the pain threshold, reduces swelling, muscle cramps and spasms.

IMPORTANT: Tien chi, safflower, rehmannia, myrrh and frankincense have very strong effects on blood flow. If taken by pregnant women, even through the skin, they can cause a miscarriage. To put it simply, they break up and sweep away blood clots; in early stages of development, a human embryo will be misidentified as a blood clot and swept away. Do not use this formulation if you are pregnant. Also, do not use "red flower oil" as a tea for colds or flu if you are pregnant.

"The body takes what it needs from a formula," Dr. Buller relates. "As long as it is reasonably balanced, it will fit several situations without creating excesses for the body to deal with. Different people have different healing capacities: even within the body, one bruise might require more of the blood invigorators (circulatory stimulants), and another bruise might require more of the painkillers. The body tends to place healing properties in order needed, as long as it is not presented with an excess in one area. For example, if I added two or three more blood invigorators, it would unbalance the formula and confuse the body.

"This is one advantage of herbal medicine," he adds. "The body can take what it needs and throw away the rest without too much trouble, since the plants have their own buffering systems. Synthetic drugs are difficult to metabolize and can stress the body if introduced in an unbalanced or excessive form."

Buying ingredients: (Stalking the savage dried herb)

It will be difficult to find most of these ingredients unless you have access to a Chinese herb shop. These can be found in most large American and Canadian cities. Your next problem will be explaining what you want. Another problem will be that some herbalists may refuse to sell you what you ask [or, simply because they're afraid you might hurt yourself.

The easiest method is to clip out the handy form with the Chinese characters accompanying the article. Ask for an ounce of each (that's also written on the page), since they may not want to bother with smaller quantities. This will give you enough to make six quarts of dit da jow. Each of these ingredients is available without a prescription.

A few blocks can make a big difference in price. While researching this article, I went to a well-stocked herbarium in the "yuppie" neighborhood or Greenwich Village, N.Y. They had most of the items, and acceptable substitutes for those they didn't have. However, they were charging $28 per ounce for **tien chi;** I had been told to expect tien chi to cost $7-8 per ounce. Buying the ingredients there would cost me over $35.

My next stop was an herbarium in the 200 block of Canal St. in the heart of Chinatown. As I started asking for different items, the herbalist eyed me with some hesitation.

"Whatcha making?" he asked.

"*Dit da jow,*" I answered, "external use only."

Apparently satisfied, he picked up a hand-held balance scale and began to measure out the ingredients. His tien chi cost $7 per ounce; the total shopping list came to $13.50. He was amused, not only by my reports of $28 tien chi, but at the sight of a six-foot, blue-eyed, red-haired **lo fan** speaking broken Chinese and gesturing wildly at his jars of dried plants. Finally, he asked to see my list, obviously deciding I'd do less damage to his language by writing it than by speaking it.

Not only did I save over $20, but I was certain I had the correct herbs - and they were fresher! Chinese herbariums usually keep the herbs in a cut-and-dried form, which makes it easier to identify the plant. Western herbariums often chop or grind the herb, so that it's easier to use, but more difficult to identify. It also tends to go stale quicker.

Remember: courtesy (attitude, attempting to learn some Chinese) can payoff in a Chinese herbarium - literally. Herbalists frequently give better prices to customers they'd like to see again. Rude people pay full list price.

Preparation

Coarsely crush each ingredient in a mortar. Grinding to powder is not as good, since the powders will form a sticky sediment which can interfere with solubility.

A word of caution about mortars: The wooden and ceramic models often found in gourmet shops are meant for crushing spices. Some of these ingredients, especially the stony *tien chi,* are just too tough. The ideal is the old apothecary-style brass mortar and pestle. Good luck finding one! The cheap substitute is a hammer and a brick. Wrap the root in denim canvas, or leather, and hit it a few times with a solid hammer. That should do the initial breaking, and you can follow up with a kitchen-type mortar if necessary.

The usual ratio is an ounce of dried plant to a pint of liquid. Place all ingredients in a one-quart bottle. Fill with a mixture of ethyl alcohol and water (80-90-proof vodka is quite good). Some of the botanical compounds are soluble in water, and some are soluble in alcohol, so the alcohol/water combination is necessary to properly dissolve them. Water or alcohol alone won't do it. Do not use methyl or isopropyl alcohol.

For the first three days, shake the mixture several times each day. This allows the water and alcohol to circulate through the ingredients. Then set the bottle in a cool, dark place, agitating it every few days.

"Synthetic drugs are difficult to metabolize and can stress the body if introduced in an unbalanced or excessive form,"
-Dr. Lyle Buller

Some herbalists believe the extended soaking period gives the botanical compounds a chance to intermingle and form new compounds, to "grow together and have offspring." When the liquid becomes opaque (in a month), it's ready to use.

Application

This dit da jow is specifically for bruises, which are primarily injuries to the blood vessels. It is not recommended for sprains, which are injuries to the muscles, or strains, which are injuries to the joint ligaments. Warm the jow in your hands, and then rub it into the affected

With that he got up, bowed and shook hands, and left to continue his daily five-mile walk. Dr. Lyle Buller, a naturopath and iron palm practitioner, explains what this formula needs to accomplish:

Jian Gu Jow 腱骨酒 Tendon & Bone Wine

"One of the first goals of iron palm training is to strengthen the tendons and bones in the hands without developing too many calluses," he says. "This must be accomplished to achieve the highest level of skill in the arts." Chinese traditional arts classify systems into three levels according to a number of factors. According to this analysis, a system which promotes heavily calloused hands is of the lowest grade, while a system which retains a completely natural-looking hand is of the highest.

"One of the key sources of strength is to have tendons and bones in the hands that are like iron," Dr. Buller explains. "This is where the power begins. Calluses themselves are useless if the tendons and bones in the hand are weak or injured. It's important to avoid injury while training, and to heal injuries as quickly as possible. If injuries to the tendons and bones are not healed correctly, the hands and forearms lose strength, flexibility and circulation. This can lead to stiffness, reduced circulation, and to symptoms like arthritis (inflamed joints), tendonitis (inflamed tendons), or rheumatism.

"This formula is based on the need to strengthen tendons and bones in the hands as well as in the joints, and to heal old injuries to these parts of the body. This formula can be used before practice for the first one-to-three months, and post-practice. The formula is warm in nature, not hot," he adds. "A hot formula can be used after the first three months, when the hands have become accustomed to the iron palm training. Also, a hot formula tends to aggravate old injuries because it concentrates on drawing out a great deal of chi, something an injured area is not prepared to handle."

Attrition because of injury is one of the greatest reasons for dropouts at martial arts schools. It's been estimated that the average school will lose 20 percent of its students in the first year because of injuries, many coming because students resume training too soon after an injury, and reinjure the same area.

"Unity of Opposites" Theory

"Yin and yang theory divides the body into the internal yin and external yang body," Dr. Buller says. The five-element theory divides each of these into five main parts corresponding to the elements of earth, metal, water, wood, and fire."

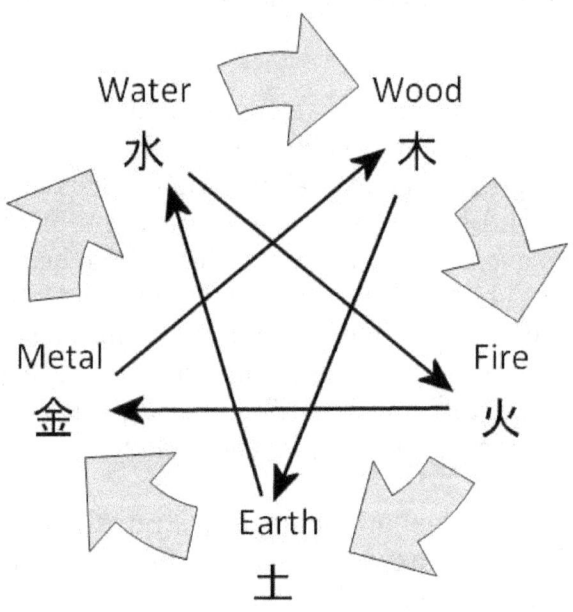

Internal body	External body
earth -pancreas	earth -muscle
metal-lung	metal-skin
water -kidney	water -bone
wood -liver	wood -tendon
fire-heart	fire-blood

The chart above shows how the Taoist concept of Five Elements relates to traditional Chinese medicine (TCM). The outer ring of arrows show which elements reinforce each other - wood feeds and supports fire, for example - while the inner pentagram shows which deconstructs another - metal (ax) deconstructs wood. Tendon and bone belong to the external yang body and are associated with wood and water elements. Therefore, theory states that strengthening the tendon and bone can be accomplished be selecting herbs which tone the wood and water elements of the external yang body.

"Also, the blood should be nourished and invigorated to maintain proper balance with the herbs that strengthen tendons and bones," Dr. Buller adds. "At the same time, toning the metal and earth elements will prevent them from being destroyed, and will regulate the wood and water elements. Earth and water mutually regulate each other, metal and wood mutually regulate each other. (Further details can be found in *The Yellow Emperor's Acupuncture Classic.*)

"Tendon and bone are located beneath the protective chi (wei chi)," Dr. Buller notes. "External pernicious influences can accumulate and stagnate in the tendons and joints when practicing, or if there is an injury. If these influences are not expelled and regulated they will impair functioning of the tendons and joints. An example of this is old injuries where the tendons and joints become stiff and painful. This is often due to stagnated chi in the tendons and joints which reduces circulation. The injury becomes stiff and painful, and sometimes feels cold."

The Herbs

杜仲	Tu Chung	*Eucommia ulmoides*
骨碎补	Ku Sui Pu	*Drynaria fortunei*
续断	Hsu Tan	*Dipsacus asper*
巴戟天	Pai Chi Tan	*Morinda officialis*
没药	Mo Yao	*Commiphora molmol*
乳香	Ru Hsiang	*Boswellia glabra*
赤芍	Chih Shao	*Paeonia rubra*
土牛膝	Niu Hsi	*Achyranthes bidentata*
黄芪	Huang Chi	*Astragalus membranecous*
熟地黄	Shu Di Huang	*Rehmannia glutinosa*
防风	Fang Feng	*Siler divaricatum*
刺五加	Wu Chia Pi	*Acanthopanax gracilistylus*

First Function: Strengthening Tendon and Bone

The primary function of this formula is to strengthen the tendons and bones of the hand and joints. This is accomplished By selecting herbs that tonify the wood and water aspects of the external yang body. Four herbs that complement each other in function and tonify the yang are used to' achieve this goal. Also, all four herbs are associated with the liver (wood, tendon) and the kidneys (water, bone), which is why they've traditionally been used for these types of injuries. Note:

The herbs will be named in Chinese, with the botanical name in parentheses, followed by common names.

杜仲 Tu Chung *(Eucommia ulmoides)* Eucommia

This is the commanding herb in this category, and is traditionally paired with ox knee, the leading herb in the next category. Together, these two herbs determine the primary nature of the formula.

"This is one of the most interesting herbs I've ever encountered," Dr. Buller comments. "The bark, which comes from a temperate-zone cousin of the rubber tree, contains a resin which can stretch like glue without breaking. When you slice this bark, the pieces are held together by the resin and the result looks something like the belly scales of a snakeskin." If the shop sells you unsliced bark, you can slice it into quarter-inch strips with a papercutter.

Tu chung, which occurs in Chinese herbal literature as early as 3,000 years ago, is also one of the herbs now under considerable scrutiny by Western pharmaceutical companies, especially for use without side effects against high blood pressure. As a result, this will be one of the more expensive herbs in the formula.

巴戟天 Pa Chi Tan *(Morinda officinalls)* Morinda

This herb looks like strips of grayish, flattened link sausage. Pat chi tan should be broken up before using.

续断 Hsu Tuan *(Dipsacus asper)* Teasel

This root bark is sold in flat slices, and it has a brownish-red appearance.

骨碎补 Ku Sui Po *(Drynaria fortunei)* Drynaria

These three herbs assist the Eucommia.

Second Function: Invigorating the blood

"With iron palm training, and especially with old injuries, it's important to invigorate the blood," Dr. Buller maintains. "The chi and the blood (fire, heart) element are the pathways between the internal yin and the external yang bodies. It's extremely important to keep them in balance, because the chi is considered primarily yang and the blood considered primarily yin. When the chi is tonified, it's sometimes necessary to tonify the blood to maintain a balance. Four herbs are compounded to achieve this effect. All are traditionally associated with the liver, which is why they have been used to invigorate the blood for injuries to the tendons."

土牛膝 Niu Hsi (*Achyrantbes bidentata*) Ox Knee
"Ox knee invigorates the blood, especially the flow of blood through the joints and tendons and it also acts to control swelling as a diuretic (an unusual combination of properties in one herb, and the reason the herb is so highly regarded). When sold in herb shops, it's usually cut into pieces about two inches long and a quarter-inch in diameter." Niu hsi promotes circulation, dissolves clots, and nourishes sinew and bones.

赤芍 Chih shao (*Paeonia rubra*) Red peony root
Three types of peony are traditionally used in Chinese medicine: red (*Paeonia rubra*), white (*Paeonia albiflora* or *lactiflora*) and tree peony (*Paeonia moutan*). In our iron palm bruise formula, white peony was used to nourish the blood. In this iron palm sinew formula, red peony is used to invigorate the blood. *Chih shao* is light red, and is usually sliced in Hong-Kong or Taiwan before shipment to America. If it's solid, slice it before using.

没药 Mo Yao (*Commiphora molmol*) Myrrh
Myrrh has been used for over 4,000 years and is one of the herbs that shows up frequently in history. The resinous

extrusion of a Middle Eastern vine, it was introduced to China by Arab physicians on trade routes from Persia and Africa. The herb sometime resembles its cousin, frankincense, The hardened sap is yellow-brown and wood-like, and crumbles under pressure.

In Chinese herbcraft, myrrh is used for almost every type of external injury associated with martial arts: bruising, fractures, sprains, and impact injuries. It was used extensively by Mongol soldiers. Myrrh improves circulation, invigorates the blood, and kills pain caused by poor circulation.

乳香 Ru Hsiang (*Boswellia glabra*) Frankincense

With a history similar to myrrh's, frankincense is always found with myrrh as a partner. Its appearance is a blue-gray to amber and translucent, with a texture like pebbles rather than wood chips. It will fracture rather than crumble under pressure. Both myrrh and frankincense should be crushed.

Third Function: Toning the Chi

Dr. Buller explains, "One herb is used to tonify the chi in a five-element approach. First, the four herbs that strengthen the yang will also tonify the chi indirectly, most notably the water and wood elements. To regulate these elements, metal and earth are tonified slightly. In a large amount, metal would destroy wood (as a landslide fills in a well). However, in small amounts metal regulates wood, and earth regulates water. Therefore, the following herb is used to tonify the chi and thereby regulate chi in injuries to tendon and bone."

黃芪 Huang Chi (Astragalus membranecous) Vetch

Called yellow vetch or milk vetch in English, it's sometimes erroneously called locoweed. True locoweeds such as datura bind selenium from the soil, causing delirium when eaten by humans. This doesn't happen with huang chi. Sometimes called "Chinese tongue depressors" because of the broad, flat appearance of sliced huang chi, it can be pricy in some neighborhoods because of claims that it strengthens the immune system against AIDS. As a result, some people are paying up to a dollar a slice of huang chi, which more realistically sells for seven-to-eight dollars a pound.

Fourth function: Toning the Blood

In most formulas that deal with injuries, it's essential to tonify the blood.

熟地黄 Shu Di Huang (Rehmannia glutinosa, steamed)

"This herb is selected because it's associated with the liver (wood, tendon) kidney (water, bone) and heart (fire, blood) systems. These qualities are why *shu di huang* is traditionally used to nourish the blood when there are also injuries to the tendons and joints. Prepared rehmannia is such a powerful herb that it's used alone in formula for this function. If additional herbs were used in this category, they would complement this herb, or accept orders from this commander, and thereby redirect the action of the entire formula. Rehmannia also nourishes the yin."

Rehmannia is the same dark, resinous root used in the iron palm bruise lotion, except that there we used it raw to cool the blood. In this sinew liniment, the prepared root is used because it nourishes the blood and yin system. The raw root is prepared by soaking and cooking in vinegar. Since you're buying this from an herbalist, it will already be prepared. Since the properties of the cooked and raw roots are different, it's essential that you keep them in separate containers and clearly labeled. Dr. Buller once learned this the hard way, and had to discard all his *di huang* because he had confused the labels and couldn't tell them apart. (Fans of kung-fu movies will know that this is one of the "secret herbs" compounded with rhinoceros horn when the hero is seriously injured, and the old master and fellow students scrape together their money to buy expensive herbs to save his life.)

Fifth Function: Expelling External Pernicious Influences

"One herb is enough to expel the BPI that enter and accumulate in the tendons after an injury," notes Dr. Buller. "One of the external influences is called wind. In the I Ching, wind is synonymous with wood as one of the eight trigrams (paqua). Wind represents movement and transformation in nature; in this instance, it's drastic change, such as hot and cold temperatures, or dry and rainy seasons. When there's an injury to the tendons, the wei chi does not function, and energy in the tendons is influenced by outside changes; the chi begins to accumulate and stagnate, which impairs tendon function. Remember, the body is subject to outside forces at all times and must be able to protect itself."

防风 Fang feng *(Siler divaricatum)* Siler

This plant is used to expel external pernicious influences from tendon and muscle. In the bruise lotion, cinnamon twigs were used to expel EPI from the wei chi itself. "If an injury is prolonged or occurs deeper than the wei chi," Dr. Buller says, "exterior chi can accumulate in the tendons and muscles. This is one of the causes of muscular aches and pain during the flu season, and when recovering from injury to the tendons." It doesn't need to be crushed; the root is yellow and usually sold in small round pieces. It's often paired in formulas with acanthopanax.

Sixth Function: "Control Wind, Expel Dampness"

The other most notable "external influence" that affects injuries to the tendons and joints is dampness. One herb is used to expel this influence. "Dampness is represented by water in the I Ching Pa Kua, and is associated with the kidney (water, bone) meridian. In the I Ching, water represents stillness, like the quiet lake; however, when the flow of water stops, the lake stagnates and begins to die. This metaphor is appropriate for the water chi in the body. Expelling the excess dampness and regulating the effect of the environment on the tendons and joint will allow them to heal more quickly," says Dr. Buller.

刺五加 Wu Chia Pi *(Acaothopanax gracilstylus)*

This herb is most suited to regulate the external pernicious influences because it is associated with both liver (wood, tendon) and kidney (water, bone) elements. This herb has been erroneously identified by some as Siberian ginseng *(eleutherococus senticoccus),* and has also been used as a substitute in products which reputedly contain Siberian ginseng. The root is solid and sold in curled gray-yellow fragments. Acanthopanax is sometimes paired with siler to protect injuries from outside influences.

Herb Summary

To strengthen tendon and bone:

Tu Chung	Eucommia ulmoides	"snakeskin"
Ku Sui Pu	Drynaria fortunei	drynaria
Hsu Tan	Dipsacus asper	teasel
Pai Chi Tan	Morinda officialis	morinda

To invigorate blood circulation:

Niu Hsi	Achyranthes bidentata	ox knee
Mo Yao	Ccommiphora molmol	myrrh
Ju Hsiang	Boswellia glabra	frankincense
Chih Shao	Paeonia rubra	red peony root

To tone and purify chi:

Huang Chi	Astragalus membranecous	yellow vetch

To tone and purify blood:

Shu Di Huang	Rehmannia glutinosa	prepared rehmannia

To expel "external pernicious influences"
Fang Feng   Siler divaricatum   siler

To regulate "external pernicious influences"
Wu Chin Pi   Acanthopanax gracilistylus

Dr. Buller notes, "Almost all of these herbs are associated with liver and kidney elements. This may sound out of balance, but this is a formula specific to the joints and tendons. One of the most important principles followed by Chinese herbalists is to nourish the liver and kidney internally because they often are prone to loss of proper function. Also, externally, it's important to maintain tendons and joints, because when a joint decreases in function, an entire section of the body can decrease in function as well."

Preparation

Do not use methyl alcohol! This is poisonous wood alcohol, and can be absorbed through the skin. Also, do not use isopropyl alcohol. This is rubbing alcohol and penetrates too deeply into the skin.

Ethyl alcohol is the type used in beverages for human consumption. (That's right, friends, we're going to rub spiced booze on ourselves again!)

Some of the active ingredients in the herbs will dissolve in alcohol, and some will dissolve in water. An almost even mixture of alcohol and water will dissolve both. Don't worry about determining this mixture yourself. The distillers have already prepared it for you -it's called cheap strong vodka.

This formula strengthens tendons in the hands and joints, while helping heal old injuries," -The author

The standard ratio is two ounces of dry herb to one quart of vodka. One-sixth ounce of each of the 12 herbs will give you a total of two ounces of herb, requiring a quart of vodka.

Place the crushed herbs in a large glass jar and pour in the vodka. Shake it gently twice a day to allow the fluid to circulate through any build-up of sediment that might form on the bottom. After six weeks, pour the liniment into smaller glass bottles, and discard the berb residue in the large jar. Do not drink the liniment! It probably won't kill you, but it can eat the lining off your stomach.

The lotion can then be used before and after iron palm practice, according to your sifu's instructions.

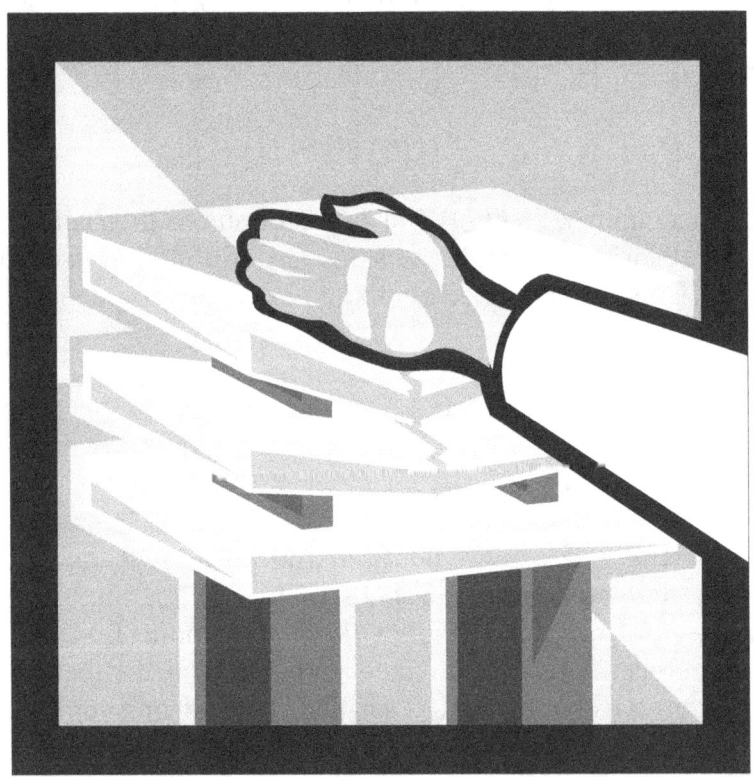

Painful Injury Powder   痛苦的傷害粉

One more formula, which was NOT part of my original series of articles with Dr. Buller. As previous mentioned, injury is the most common reason beginning martial artists quit. Impact, overexertion, overextension - there are any number of reasons. This is one of the classical formulations.

Herb Summary by Function:

To Tonify Chi and Blood:
人参 Ren Shen   (Panax ginseng)

To Invigorate Blood and Resolving Stagnation:
琥珀 Hu Po   (Amber)

To Promoting the Flow of Chi, to Reduce Pain and Swelling, and to Promote Tissue Regeneration:
乳香 Ru Xiang   (Frankincense)
没药 Mo Yao   (Myrrh)

To Promote Tissue Regrowth and Heal Wounds:
珍珠 Zhen Zhu   (Freshwater pearl)

To Eliminate Stagnation and Stop Bleeding:
血竭 Xue Jie (Dragon's Blood resin -*Daemonorops draco blume*)

To Tonify and Invigorate Blood:
当归 Dang Gui   (Angelica sinensis)

To Stop Bleeding and Relieve Stagnation:
田七 Tien Chi   (Notoginseng)

To Clear "Heat" and Reduce Pain.
龙脑 Bing Pian   (Camphor resin)

To Refreshing the Mind and Reduce Pain:
麝香 She Xiang   (Dwarf Deer Musk)

To Clear "Heart-Fire" and Reduce Toxicity.
牛黄 Niu Huang   (Cow or Deer gallstone)

This formula is traditionally ground into a fine powder and applied externally in coconut oil or a similar carrier. It can also be prepared in advance by soaking the powdered ingredients for at least a week in a mixture of water and alcohol, such as vodka.

Three Formulas

If you have access to a Chinese apothecary shop, just photocopy this page and hand it to the herbalist like a prescription.

Dit Da Bruise Lotion

Please give me one ounce of each:
請給我1盎司各:

1. **桂枝**　　Gui Zhi　　(Cinnamomum cassia)
2. **生地黃**　Sheng di huang (raw Rehmannia glutinosa)
3. **藕根**　　Lien tzu　　(Nelumbo nucifera)
4. 田七　　Tien chi　　(Panax notoginseng)
5. **黃芩**　　Huang sun　(Scutellaria baicalensis)
6. **红花**　　Hung hua　　(Carthamus tinctorus)
7. 乳香　　Ru Hsiang　(Boswellia glabra)
8. 没药　　Mo yao　　(Commiphora maImaI)
9. **川芎**　　Chuan Xiong (Ligusticum lucidum/wallachii)
10. **甘草**　Kan tsao　　(Glycyrrhizae uralensis)
11. **当归**　Tang kuei　(Angelicae sinensis)
12. 白芍　　Pai shao　　(Paeonia albiflora)

谢谢!　Thank you!

If you have access to a Chinese apothecary shop, just photocopy this page and hand it to the herbalist like a prescription.

Dit Da Joint and Tendon Lotion

Please give me one ounce of each:
請給我1盎司各:

1. **杜仲**   Tu Chung   *(eucommia ulmoides)*
2. 骨碎补   Ku Sui Pu   *(drynaria fortunei)*
3. 续断   Hsu Tan   *(dipsacus asper)*
4. **巴戟天**   Pai Chi Tan *(morinda officialis)*
5. **没药**   Mo Yao   *(commiphora molmol)*
6. **乳香**   Ru Hsiang   *(boswellia glabra)*
7. **赤芍**   Chih Shao   *(Paeonia rubra)*
8. **土牛膝**   Niu Hsi   *(achyranthes bidentata)*
9. **黄芪**   Huang Chi   *(astragalus membranecous)*
10. **熟地黄** Shu Di Huang *(rehmannia glutinosa)*
11. **防风**   Fang Feng   *(siler divaricatum)*
12. **刺五加** Wu Chia Pi   *(acanthopanax gracilistylus)*

谢谢!   Thank you!

If you have access to a Chinese apothecary shop, just photocopy this page and hand it to the herbalist like a prescription.

Painful Injury Powder　痛苦的傷害粉

Please assemble the following ingredients in the amounts indicated, ground into a fine powder
請聚集在指定的金額，地面以下成分成細粉

人参 Ren Shen 1.5 g　　　(Panax ginseng)

珍珠 Zhen Zhu 1.5 g　　　(Freshwater pearl)

琥珀 Hu Po 1.5 g　　　(Amber)

当归 Dang Gui 1.5 g　　　(Angelica sinensis)

龙脑 Bing Pian 1.5 g　　　(Camphor resin)

乳香 Ru Xiang 1.5 g　　　(Frankincense)

没药 Mo Yao 1.5 g　　　(Myrrh)

田七 Tien Chi 1.5 g　　　(Notoginseng)

血竭 Xue Jie 6 g　　　(Dragon's Blood resin)

麝香 She Xiang 0.9 g　　　(Dwarf Deer Musk)

牛黄 Niu Huang 0.3 g　　　(Cow or Deer gallstone)

谢谢！　Thank you!

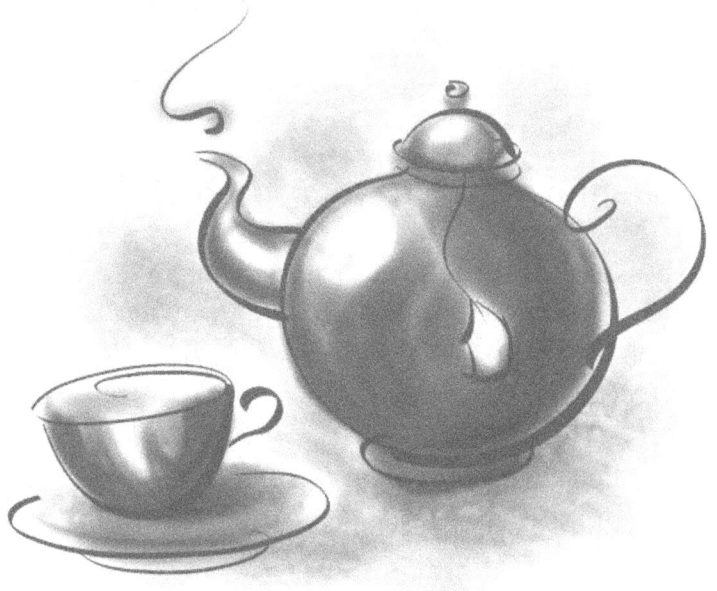

Energy Teas: Charge Up with Just a Cup!

Homemade Chinese teas can help you wake up and bulk up without all those nagging side effects.

There comes a time in everyone's training when you want a little more energy. How can you wisely use herbs without spending hours at the herbal medicine books? How can you "bulk up" without the harmful side effects of steroids and other synthetic chemicals?

Each of these formulas has a long and successful association with martial arts, and is noted for a lack of harmful effects,

#1 Kung-Fu Tea

Equal weights of:

黨參	tang shen	*Codonopsis lanceolate*
白朮	pai shu	*Atractylus ovata*
茯苓	fu ling	*Poria cocos*
甘草	kan tsao	*Glycyrrhizae uralensis*
蜂蜜	feng mi	Honey (to taste)

This is a rather common formula in China, and has the advantages of low cost and simplicity. ***Tang shen*** is a long root, looking somewhat like shriveled ginseng roots or a cross between ginseng and unpainted pencils. It's often used instead of real ginseng for young men, since it won't produce an excess of yang energy known as "false fire," which can result in headaches and irritability. Some herb dealers have even tried to pass off *tang shen* as ginseng to less-experienced customers.

A pound of each ingredient should cost no more than $40 total. One of the easiest ways I've found to brew these-teas is to p1ace the dry ingredients in the glass pot of a drip coffeemaker, and let the boiling water drip onto them. The beating element then keeps the pot on a very low simmer, so the brew gets stronger. After one to two hours, it'll be surprisingly strong. Just strain the mixture through a tea strainer.

Ginseng and Reality

Since each of these following formulas uses ginseng, let's start with a little background on this highly prized and often overpriced herb.

"Ginseng" is a generic name for a wide variety of related plants found in Asia and North America, mostly of the botanical family Aralia. Their common characteristic is a knobby "man-shaped" root with a slightly sweet flavor. The varieties of "ginseng" and some of its close cousins are:

Panax ginseng mei
Chinese/Korean ginseng
Panax quinquefolium
American (five-leafed) ginseng
Panax trifolium
American dwarf ginseng
Panax pseudoginseng (aka **panax notoginseng, Panax bipinnatifidum**)
San chi, tien chi, prince ginseng, Himalayan ginseng
Panax japonica
Japanese ginseng
Eleutherococcus senticocus
Siberian Ginseng
Acanthopanax gracistylus (aka **eleutherococcus gracistylus**)
Wu Ji Pia
Codonopsis lanceolate
Tang shen, "poor man's ginseng"

Related North American medicinal plants:

Caulophyllum thalictroides
Blue cohosh
Triosteum perfoliatum
Fever root
Aralia nudicaulis
Wild or Virginia Sarsaparilla,
Aralia hispida
Bristly Sarsaparilla
Aralia racemosa
American Spikenard

Each plant has a different use and is surrounded by its own lore. For example, **Panax ginseng** comes in several grades with names such as "heaven," "earth," "unicorn," and the wild *"tung pei."* The difference in grades can be drastic in effect and price.

Panax quinquefolium L . - **American "Five-Leaf" Ginseng**
Considered to be more "yang" in its makeup than the Chinese. variety, and was in demand by Chinese herbalists when more "yang" was called for; American trader John Jacob Astor made a fortune shipping American ginseng to China in return for Chinese tea -and almost exterminated the species by overharvesting.

E. senticocus - Siberian Ginseng
This has been used by Soviet Olympic athletes and cosmonauts for its stamina-building properties, and is said to relieve arthritis pain.

Panax pseudoginseng -
Supposedly part of the cure used by the rustic Russian monk Grigory Rasputin to control the hemophilia of Prince Alexei. Some call it prince ginseng as a result. **Tienchi** is also an ingredient in the famed patent medicine **Yunnan Bai Yao,** used for severe wounds by all sides in the Vietnam War. **Yunnan Bai Yao** has also been popular with martial artists who use bladed weapons!

Ginseng formulas are best taken on an empty stomach, when the expensive ginseng doesn't have to fight other foods for absorption. Some herbalists advise you to wait three hours after taking ginseng before eating acid fruits such as citrus.

Also, ginseng should not be brewing in a ferrous container. Glass, porcelain, or ceramic is preferred, since metals can interact with components of the ginseng to produce unwanted compounds.

How much will ginseng cost? The better grades (*yi sun, tung pei*) can cost $50 per ounce and more. The lower grades (*kirin*; lower quality *shiu chu*) will cost $4-$5 per ounce. The age, size, and growing conditions of the ginseng also affect prices. I've personally found $10-$15 per-ounce, 7-year-old forest-grown American ginseng (shaken, not stirred) to be just fine. This is something like buying fine wines: if you don't know why this bottle costs more, you're probably better off with something cheaper.

I've also found both tang shen and sarsaparilla to be worthwhile low-budget substitutes.

#2 Kung-Fu Tea

This tea is associated with the martial artist who wants to "bulk up," building both muscle and stamina. It's more drastic in its effect, and costs quite a bit more. Good ginseng will cost at least $7-$10 an ounce.

Equal weights of (no common English name for some):

ren shen	*Panax ginseng*	ginseng
huang chi	*Astragalus membranecous*	vetch
pai shu	*Atractylis ovata*	n/a
chai hu	*Bupleurum falcatum*	Sickle leaf hare's ear
chen pi	*Citrus aurantia*	orange peel
kan chiang	*Zingiber officialis*	ginger
ta tsao	*Jujube sinensis*	red date
kan tsao	*Glycyrrhizae uralensis*	licorice

#3 Ginseng Tea

A popular way of enjoying ginseng. Some prefer to leave out the ginger, since its strong taste easily overpowers the delicate taste of the ginseng. The ginger and licorice add an immediate energy boost, while the ginseng's power kicks in slowly. Some also add a slight bit of clove.

Equal weights of:

ren shen	*Panax ginseng*	ginseng
kan chiang	*Zingiber officialis*	ginger
kuei pi	*Cinnamomum cassia*	cinnamon
kan tsao	*Glycerrhizae uralensis or glabra*	licorice
chen pi	*Citrus aurantium*	orange peel

In teas that contain cinnamon, the cinnamon is added 20 to 30 minutes before taking the tea off the heat.

#4 Sentry's Tea

Equal weights of:

ren shen	*Panax ginseng*	ginseng
kuei pi	*Cinnamomum* cassia	cinnamon
kan tsao	*Glycyrrhizae uralensis*	licorice
shih hu	*Dendobrium hancockii*	orchid stem

Half as much of:

ma huang	*Ephedra sinensis*	ephedra

According to legend, this formula was given to Genghis Khan's sentries so they could stay alert all night. ***Ma huang*** is a potent stimulant, and should be used in small quantities. It's also used to clear phlegm from the lungs, so don't be surprised if you start coughing up mucous. Sentry tea has been used by students cramming their way through "all-nighters," and as an aid to meditation. If the effects are too stimulating, decrease or eliminate the *ma huang.* NOTE: The FDA banned ephedra as a food ingredient

A warning: stimulant teas are no substitute for sleep. Don't rely on this for long-distance driving. When it wears off, it does so suddenly, and you'll find yourself as fatigued as you really should be. As with caffeine products such as coffee, coffee syrup candy, and guarana, they should be considered "fatigue maskers" rather than "stimulants."

#5 Lenape Spring Tonic

Equal weights of:

ginseng	*Panax quinquefoliurn or trifolium*
sarsapanlla	*Aralia nudicaulis*
licorice	*Glycerrhizae glabra*
false spikenard	*Smilacina racemosa*
burdock root	*Arctium lappa or minus*
birch bark	*Betula lenta*
cherry bark	*Prunus serotina*
motherwort	*Leonurus cardiaca*
dandelion	*Taraxacum officinalis*
boneset	*Eupatorium perfoliatum*
sassafras root	*Sassafras officinalis*
sweetflag	*Acorus calamus*

This tea was popular with the Lenape (Delaware) tribe, who ranged from the Hudson Valley to the Chesapeake, and was used as a nutrient-rich food in the spring to make up for months of a nutrient-poor winter diet of game and preserved food.

Ginseng, burdock, dandelion, sarsaparilla, licorice and boneset are **alteratives**, a class of herbs which detoxify and normalize the entire system. Dandelion is one of the best high-nutrient, high-fiber, low-calorie foods available, and it grows wild in most of North America. The entire plant can be used, or just dried root. Boneset and motherwort are dried leaves, the other ingredients are roots.

Sweetflag and sassafras are added to the brew in the final 15-20 minutes, since they are quite strong and can make the brew taste gummy if cooked for too long. Do not use sassafras leaves, or you'll end up with a gelatinous mess that won't even pour.

Conclusion

The most important thing to remember when using herbal approaches is consistency. You can't use herbal supplements the way TV commercials promote Western pharmaceuticals: a few drops or pills, and in just seconds you get fast, fast relief. Herbal teas must be used several times each day, and it may take a few weeks before you notice the effects. Be patient with yourself, and take some consolation from the fact that each of these formulations tastes pretty good.

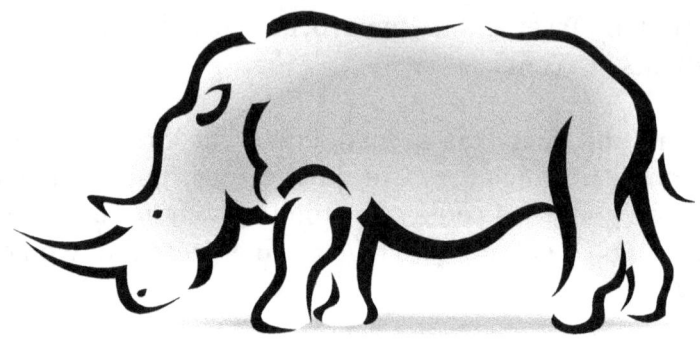

Farewell, Rhinoceros Horn

In my younger days, Manhattan's Chinatown was a wonderland of the exotic! It was an explosion of sights, smells, colors, and tastes. The windows of the Chinese, Korean, and later Vietnamese apothecaries were full of strange ingredients. Whole, dried geckos flattened out and poised like flying dinosaurs... ginseng roots that looked like sculptures... antlers and spiral horns that looked like they came from unicorns... dried snakes and sea creatures defying description. But perhaps the most exotic, and in hindsight sad, was rhinoceros horn.

To be fair, I came to realize that "rhinoceros horn" was more likely to be dark slices of rehmannia and other herbs resembling cross-sections of horn or antlers, placed and labeled to prank or shock the tourist. The real rhino horn was powdered and kept behind the counter for up to $2,000 an ounce.

But all that has changed, and the rhino horn is gone.

Four rhino species and one subspecies are protected as endangered under the U.S. Endangered Species Act. This law makes it illegal to import or export rhino and rhino parts and products; it also prohibits interstate commerce. Rhinos are also protected globally under the Convention on International Trade in Endangered Species.

These animals face extinction in part because of the world's longstanding lust for their horn, which has been valued for centuries as a carving material and medicinal.

Rhino horn is made up primarily of keratin – a protein found in hair, fingernails, and animal hooves. When carved and polished, horn takes on a translucence and luster that increase as the object ages.

In ancient Greece, rhino horn was believed to have the ability to purify water. Persians in the 5th century B.C. thought that rhino horn vessels could be used to detect poisoned liquids, which would bubble when poured into such cups. Many cultures at times shared this belief, as did the crowned heads of Europe up through the 18th and 19th centuries. And, in fact, chemists have concluded that there may be some truth in the theory – if the poisons happen to be alkaloids, which might react with the keratin in the rhino horn.

Artisans in China used rhino horn for ornamentation as long ago as the 7th century. For hundreds of years, it was customary for Chinese nobles to mark the emperor's birthday with the gift of a carved rhino horn drinking cup.

Museums and private collectors worldwide prize these antiques for both their beauty and monetary value.

In Yemen, rhino horn was long used for making the handles of special curved daggers that are presented to adolescent boys as a sign of manhood and devotion to Islam.

The ornamental application of rhino horn was a "high society" decorative "fad" in Europe in the late 19th and early 20th centuries. Through the 1920s, items made from horn ranged from walking sticks and door handles to pistol grips and limousine interiors.

The medicinal use of rhino horn also dates back centuries. Medical practitioners in such Asian countries as Malaysia, Korea, Vietnam, India and China used it as a treatment for many different symptoms and illnesses. In traditional Chinese medicine, ground rhino horn was prescribed for lowering fever and ameliorating such disorders as rheumatism and gout.

Other uses in traditional medicine included treating snakebite, boils, food poisoning, and possession by spirits as well as curing headaches, hallucinations, high blood pressure, and typhoid.

Scientists have little evidence to support belief in the medical efficacy of rhino horn, and many practitioners of traditional medicine have stopped using it in light of the species' plight. Yet such belief persists and is fueled by "urban legends" old or new about its powers as an aphrodisiac or cure for cancer.

Medicinal use continues to create demand for rhino horn – a demand that poses a threat to the continued survival of rhino species in the wild.

I never used rhino horn personally, and do not regret its ban in the slightest. However.... I did develop a taste of Three Snakes Wine... a strong rice wine containing the bile and venom of cobra, krait, and viper.

Cheers!

ABOUT THE AUTHOR

Brian Wilkes began his study of Asian martial arts in 1968. In the 1980's he became a frequent writer on the subject, with his work published in all the major martial arts publications of the time as well as an interviewer on a nationally distributed TV program, *The Martial Arts World.*

Today, he is a consultant and publisher who pursues the health benefits of the arts. This book grew from a series of articles first published in *Inside Kung Fu* magazine.

www.ingramcontent.com/pod-product-compliance
Lightning Source LLC
Chambersburg PA
CBHW070339290526
45791CB00003B/1399